Sex Guide:

Proven Tips For Mindblowing Orgasms

Table of content

Introduction

Sex is one of the most sought out, and thought about, activities throughout the world, and it has been since time began.

Physical intimacy is the most exquisite way to bond with your partner, if you are doing it right, that is. But it is so much more than just a great pastime with your lover. It is actually one of the most important activities you can do for your own wellbeing.

You may be surprised to learn that sex is an important way to stay healthy. The "WOW Orgasms: A Sex Guide to Make a Pleasure Explosion in Bed" will teach you just how important sex is for your mental, emotional and physical health. And, that is just the tip of the iceberg of what this short, yet information packed guide is going to teach you!

Before we get started, it is important to take a minute to realize how everyone knows that good sex just feels awesome! Who doesn't love to be touched, just the right way, and end up with orgasms that feel as if the earth is moving under the bed?

Thinking about how great sex is, you will learn just how truly incredible it really is because this guide will help you learn how to take sex into the realms that surpass your ultimate fantasies. It doesn't even matter how experienced or good your partner is at sex, because he or she will quickly figure out how to join you in your newfound, greatly increased performance.

Make no mistake, the best sex is going to require a bit of time and effort on your behalf. But who cares, when you are having the time of your life experiencing orgasms that will be imprinted in your memory as being the best things that ever happened to you?

In this regard, the time and effort you put into increasing the joy in your sex life is going to be more than well worth it, it might be the best thing you ever do for yourself and your partner.

This guide to WOW Sex is going to take you step by step through how to get yourself ready for the best experiences imaginable. You will learn how the actual act of sex is simply one part of the whole sexual experience. You will also learn some secret orgasm techniques that will make it possible to prolong and intensify your orgasms for absolutely explosive experiences!

Whether you are newly active with your sexual partner, or want to learn ways to spice up a long term relationship, you will learn a great deal from this guide. You may never look at sex the same way again, and you must be forewarned, it may be hard to wipe that secretive smile off your face from all the pleasure you are about to experience!

Let's get started...

Chapter 1 – The Importance of Sex

Everyone knows that sex feels great and is also how babies are made. Not so many people realize just how important having sex is for good health and wellbeing though. In fact, if more people knew how important sex was for the health, more people would be having it more often, and we would probably have much healthier communities.

Health Benefits of Sex:

-   Having sex three or more times per week reduces heart attacks and strokes by half in men, according to 2001 follow-on to the Queens University.

-   Having sex at least once a month boosts the immunity system by increasing the level of immunoglobulin A according to research conducted by Wilkes University.

-   Vigorous sex is equivalent to running for 15 minutes on a treadmill in regard to offering important cardio activity. It also burns around 200 calories.

- Levels of testosterone are increased, which creates stronger muscles and bones.

- Endorphin chemicals are released, which alleviates depression and promotes happier moods.

- Oxytocin in the body increases up to five times its normal level to relieve pain, including pain from arthritis and headaches.

- Estrogen is released in women that helps to reduce PMS symptoms. It also provides smooth skin and shiny hair.

- Reduces blemishes, suffering from dermatitis and skin rashes by providing healthy pores.

- Releases pheromones that are natural attractants.

- DHEA increases up to five times the normal level. This hormone is associated with enhanced libido, building muscles, warding off depression and aiding in a long life.

- Zinc, calcium, plasma, and other minerals in seminal plasma gives you healthier teeth and retard tooth decay during oral sex.

- Men in their twenties can reduce risks of prostate cancer by one-third by ejaculating more than five times a week according to the British Journal of Urology International.

- Acts a natural antihistamine which helps you breathe better and also combats asthma and hay fever.

- Is ten times more effective than Valium, with zero side effects.

Aside from improving your personal health on mental, emotional and physical levels, it improves the relationship with your partner. Couples who make sex an important part of their lives are happier together and less likely to split-up.

For the best results, if you are a woman, have sex as often as you like. If you are a man under the age of 29, have sex up to five times per week, and up to three to four times per week after that. More than that is not healthy for you, although occasionally having more sex per week is not going to hurt you.

If you are afraid that you will lose a sense of romance or spontaneity if you schedule sex, do not worry about it. Just schedule sex for two to three times a week. Knowing you are going to have sex will create more excitement as you look forward to it. You can still have spontaneous sex once or twice a week as well.

Chapter 2 – The WOW Sex Workout

Hearing the word workout might be off-putting, because, who wants to spend time exercising when they could be having the best sex of their lives? At the same time, there are very specific exercises which are going to have a dramatic impact on how much pleasure you will be able to receive. Not to worry, they will not take up a great deal of your time or money.

It is important to understand that sex is an endurance sport. If you are out of shape, then you are not going to be able to keep up very well. Sure, sex will still feel good, but if you want it to feel incredibly blissful, with incredibly strong orgasms, then this WOW sex workout is for you.

Both men and women should get at least twenty minutes of cardio per day in order to build the stamina for intense sex. How you get that cardio activity is up to you. If you are out of shape, start with three minutes per day and build up to the full twenty minutes.

Cardio Activities:

- Sex (of course!)

- Dancing

- Swimming

- Running

- Brisk walking

- Bicycling

- Jumping Jacks

- Aerobics

The next set of exercises you want to do are called Kegels. This is an activity where you will be squeezing genital muscles. To find the right muscles to work out for Kegel exercises, try to cut your urination off in midstream. Then, daily, start to squeeze those muscles, hold them as tightly as possible for three seconds, then relax them. Start off with three sets of three at different times of the day and build up to three sets of ten per day.

Finally, creating flexibility is going to give your sex life a fresh breath of life in huge ways. You could do simple stretching exercises, such a touching your toes. Ideally, you will want to do Yoga. Not only will Yoga increase your flexibility, it will increase your blood flow and help you become more mindful. Overall, it is a perfect recipe that will benefit your ability for increased pleasure from foreplay to completion.

Try these yoga poses:

Cat and Cow:

- Start on all fours with your shoulders directly above your wrists and your hips over your knees.

- Allow your back to push down toward the floor and lift your chest and heart away from your belly, while reaching your tailbone toward the sky.

- Push back, belly, and tailbone downward as you lower your head toward the floor.

- Repeat slowly, five times.

Bound Angle Pose

- Lay on your back

- Place the soles of your feet together by allowing knees to drop open and toward the floor.

- Relax in this position and allow the knees to drop closer and closer toward the floor for up to five minutes.

Bridge Pose

- While still lying on your back from the Bound Angle Pose:

- Place feet flat on the floor, at shoulder's distance apart, beneath your buttocks.

- Push hips toward the sky and place hands together, underneath your body, behind your back.

- Hold this pose for up to 10 breaths.

You can find other yoga poses by attending local classes, or looking up poses online, but these three poses will get you started. Each one of them has specific benefits that will help increase your sexual pleasure and lead to very strong orgasms.

Chapter 3 – The WOW Sex Diet

The WOW sex diet has nothing to do with eating to lose weight, although, if you are eating an unhealthy diet and start focusing on eating to gain sexual pleasure, you may shed a few pounds as a side effect. However, this diet is more about eating to increase your sexual potency and promote lustier sex and stronger orgasms.

Everyone knows that junk food is unhealthy and should be avoided, and that holds true if you are looking for out of this world, exquisite, sexual experiences as well. Foods that are processed, pre-packaged or loaded with chemicals and pesticides contain dead calories that take the life out of you as well. In other words, there is absolutely nothing sexy about them.

Ditch the junk and opt for wholesome, natural foods. This is especially important if you know you will be having sex within a 12 to 24 hour time period of eating. Surprisingly, though, you also want to avoid eating too many raw foods, such as salad right before having sex. Even though these foods are healthy, many types of raw vegetables create flatulence, and as you can imagine, that is not so sexy either.

Speaking of foods to avoid right before sex, anything that causes you to bloat is best avoided. Caffeinated beverages, foods with artificial sweeteners, foods containing wheat, beans and anything else that you know will cause your belly to feel too full needs to be avoided when you want to feel your sexiest ever. The sexier you feel, the better your opportunities for super orgasms.

Steamed vegetables are your best choice, and protein. Protein is a building block that will add stamina and strength. That is a much sexier way to get the full pleasure from your sexual adventures. Here are some additional foods that you will want to have on hand to help ramp up the orgasmic experiences you are searching for:

- Dark Chocolate boosts endorphins and helps to create euphoric feelings, it also increases your energy level. Do not gorge yourself on it though, a little goes a long way.

- Consider melting that dark chocolate and add a dash of red hot chili peppers, or cayenne pepper. The capsaicin will increase the blood flow in your genitals and stimulate your nerve endings.

- For extra potency, add a tiny bit of Saffron. This is an expensive spice, but it will further increase the blood flow to your genital region. It will also reduce anxiety and let's face it, feeling stressed is not going to allow you to fully surrender into the full throws of passion that will create the best orgasms ever.

- Now, dip small wedges of watermelon into the dark chocolate. The watermelon contains citrulline. This ingredient will relax the blood vessels to give you stronger erections, including for erectile tissues in the woman's clitoris and for the man's penis.

- Adding a protein source alongside of your super-sex fondue will increase your potency, but you want to avoid heavier proteins such as red meat. Instead, opt for some oysters or other type of shellfish for the best results, such as clams, mollusks, crab or lobster. These will release of surge of sex hormones, making it all the better to reach mind-blowing orgasms.

Believe it or not, alcohol or other mind altering substances should be avoided, or at least minimized. For instance, one glass of red wine may help you relax and get into a better mood for sex, but too much will numb your body and not allow you to gain the full enjoyment of your climax.

Drinking enough water is actually your best choice of beverages, and perhaps one cup of coffee or green tea. The added caffeine, in a minimal quality can help boost your energy level, and for the most satisfying sexual activities, the added energy can be helpful.

Chapter 4 – The WOW Sex Mindset

As you are preparing your body to reach the ultimate orgasms, you cannot forget about your mind. Your mind holds the key to how fully you can immerse yourself into the sexual experience, or not. Achieving the WOW sex mindset is going to take you from enjoying sex to feeling as if it has completely transported you into new dimensions of bliss.

Consider the elements of the WOW Sex mindset and start to pursue these elements in order to get your mind ready for the best sex of your life.

The Elements of the WOW Sex Mindset:

A sense of humor. While you may be very serious about wanting to experience the ultimate orgasm, if you cannot lighten up and have some fun, you will be too tense to reach the height of pleasure. Increase your laughter quotient daily for best results, including the ability to laugh at yourself. Pursue comedies, funny Facebook posts or whatever helps you laugh out loud.

A sense of experimentation. Seeking the ultimate climax is going to require an open mind and willingness to experiment. For instance, you may not reach the ultimate orgasm through missionary position sex. For you it might be through some other sexual activity. Pursue adventures by trying new sexual techniques and positions.

A sense of worthiness. No matter what, you, and everyone else, deserves the best in life. If you are feeling as if you are not enough, such as not good enough or experienced enough to reach a completely satisfying orgasm, then you will not achieve it. Pursue activities that will raise your sense of self-worth for the best results.

A sense of generosity. Unless you are masturbating, your partner deserves your complete presence during times of intimacy. Aim for pleasing your partner, while you also enjoy the sensual delights for yourself. Pursue giving to your partner without expecting anything in return sometimes.

A sense of sexiness. Consider what turns you on, and pursue that. Believe it or not, porn can be a turn on but too much of it will de-sensitize you, so use that sparingly. Find other ways to get turned on, such as fantasizing about you and your partner and visualizing what you believe the ultimate orgasm is going to feel like.

A sense of awareness. If you are worried about the bills, the kids, or your job, in the middle of having sex, then you are going to miss out on the sexiest nuances. Pursue mindfulness activities such as meditation or yoga in order to strengthen your powers of remaining in the present moment.

Chapter 5 – The WOW Sex Advanced Self-Care

At this point, you know about how to use food and exercise to get ready for the most powerful orgasms of your life. You also know that WOW starts in the mind. Now, it's time to take care of yourself, in the WOW Sex way! When it comes to this superior style of sensuality, there is no such thing as selfish. Instead, there is only the type of self-care that you pursue when you feel perfectly worthy of the best in life.

Are you wondering if you are worthy to get the absolute best of sex, and everything else in life? Well, many people struggle to feel as if they are "enough". If you struggle too, just start "faking it until you make it". That means, just start taking exquisite care of yourself, regardless of whether you feel worth it or not. Your feelings can catch up later.

Toiletry is a given, because no one wants to have sex with someone that has body odor or smelly breath. Take care of the basics, then take it a step further by creating an at home spa for yourself. You can do this on your own, or with your lover, and this is for both men and women.

At Home Spa Treatment:

Before getting started with this spa treatment, get rid of all the excess body hair. Trim, shave, pluck, or wax, whatever works best for you. Also, trim your fingernails and toenails.

1. Wash hair and massage a half cup of pure honey into your hair, wrap in a towel or plastic wrap.

2. Soak for 20 minutes in a warm bath that has 2 cups Epsom salt, 4 sprigs of fresh rosemary and a handful of fresh mint.

3. Scrub body all over with a mixture of honey and sugar (Enough sugar in the honey to form a paste). Include your face in this scrub down.

4. Before rinsing the honey-sugar scrub, place 2 cold, used tea bags or 2 cucumber slices over your eyes. Sit back in the tub and think sexy thoughts for five to ten minutes.

5. Rinse hair and body with lukewarm to cool water and massage mineral oil, or coconut oil, into your skin, instead of lotion, it will not leave a bad taste in your partner's mouth.

Removing excess hair, soaking your skin and then exfoliating it will heighten your sensitivity to your partner's touch. The Epsom salt will relax your muscles while the Rosemary and mint will enliven your mind. Overall, a complete recipe to get your body ready for the most pleasure you can possibly experience.

Chapter 6 – The WOW Sex Foreplay

The secret to effective foreplay, that most people are missing out on, is that it starts long before you take your clothes off. It starts with teasing, flirting and romance, with your partner, and with yourself. Yes, you can tease and flirt with yourself by taking extra time on your appearance and surrounding yourself with sensual experiences.

Foreplay is not about grabbing each other and going for the orgasm right away. Rather, foreplay is slow, tantalizing and is about fully experiencing each other, and your own senses. For WOW Sex foreplay, it is meant to relax the mind and body, while also creating deep desire.

When you get into the bedroom, undress each other and really take your time to get into the present moment. This is not a time to think about bills, work or anything other than enjoying the present set of circumstances, which include two naked bodies. Touch each other, slowly, gently and in a way that promotes relaxation, the excitement will build up later.

Make sure to talk to each other and let one another know what feels best. Since everyone is different, knowing how to touch each other is the beginning of the best sex ever. There is no reason to be shy with one another, because there is no shame in being honest about what feels best. There is also no judgment because people cannot really help if their body likes soft caresses, or heavier manhandling.

It can be extremely sensual to ask each other, "Does this feel good?" So ask questions and do it in an open minded way of exploration. Also, do not be shy about using lube or other sexual enhancers. In fact, for many women, complete pleasure is impossible without a vibrator because of how it stimulates to the level that her complex body requires.

For a few, super-secret WOW Sex foreplay tips:

- Use your mouth more than your tongue, and use your mouth abundantly all over your partner's body.

- Be playful, it is called fore-PLAY. When you get too serious you will both tense up and that will not promote the type of orgasm that you want.

- Build, Rest, Repeat. That means, build an excitement level to where you think you are both going to explode, but then stop. After a brief rest, not long enough to lose interest, but long enough to calm down sufficiently, repeat by starting slowly to rebuild the passion, through touching, oral sex, or through other stimulation.

The actual sex act is the final act in foreplay and should be left until you have each build up, rested and repeated at least one or two times. For the best results, try to build up to three Build, Rest, Repeat cycles.

Chapter 7 – The WOW Sex Secret Orgasm Techniques

The orgasm is the happy ending to the story of all the hard work you have been doing. To reach a WOW Orgasm, the type that rocks your whole body and leaves you feeling as if you melted, but are also empowered, is not just about stimulating your genitals. It is a celebration of all of your senses.

To start experiencing the WOW orgasm, take at least 3 to 4 weeks to follow all of the suggestions you have learned so far, including eating right, exercising, taking the ultimate care of yourself and of course, having sex. Then, stop having sex for 3 days, but continue to follow all the other suggestions.

Start with what you have learned about the WOW foreplay and allow your desire and excitement to build slowly. Also, use the Build, Rest, Repeat formula to build up to the most explosive orgasm.

WOW Orgasm Positions:

You will find the best orgasms through either the missionary, or traditional sex position, with the man on top. For women, sometimes it is best if you are on top, or in doggy style in order to get the angle and stimulation you need.

For Mind-blowing WOW Orgasms:

- Pay attention to erogenous zones, in particular, stimulating the woman's clitoris, using a vibrator or your fingers is going to help her reach the most profound orgasms.

- For men, do not be afraid to ask your partner to stroke your testicles or massage your perineum when you are getting close to the final orgasm.

- When you build, rest, and repeat, use the rest time to imagine all the sexual tension is getting absorbed into the rest of your body. Take some deep breaths, squeeze all the muscles in your body and then relax them. Get to the point where you are almost not excited anymore, but still excited enough to perform.

- Do not concentrate or worry. When you have decided that you are done with the Build, Rest, Repeat cycles, then just completely relax and enjoy the moment. Allow yourself to get completely carried away with the sensations.

- Use enough lubricant to feel comfortable, but not so much that you are slipping and sliding off of one another.

- Use toys if they help you. Vibrators are especially important for women because many of them need the intense stimulation. This does not mean there is anything wrong with their partner's performance, it is just how some women's bodies are designed. So, do not be shy about using them.

You can use a vibrator in and around the vaginal area at the same time you are having intercourse.

- For some couples, oral sex will offer the strongest orgasm, or genital massage using fingers and/or a vibrator. For this reason, take your time with different types of stimulation, outside of intercourse.

- Whether slow, gentle movements, or deep, passionate, faster movements will bring the best orgasm is up to you and your partner to figure out. Each body is different, so what works for you will be left for experimentation.

It may take a while for you and your partner to find the type of position and stimulation that invokes the most powerful orgasms. That is no problem though, because there is a great deal of pleasure to be found in every adventure.

Chapter 8 – The WOW Sex Pillow Talk

While you are experimenting with different types of stimulation, it is essential to communicate with each other. Your partner cannot read your mind, and there is no shame in asking to be touched in certain ways, in certain places. Of course, continually issuing orders, "harder, softer, faster, slower, or touch me 'here'" can cause a loss in pleasure. On the other hand, saying, "Oh baby that feels good, do it more....," can increase pleasure.

The WOW Sex pillow talk is all about building your partner up by encouraging, complimenting, and using positive requests for your own satisfaction. If you do not like what is happening, use an "I want" statement. For instance, if your partner is being too rough, avoid saying, "Ouch, you idiot, that hurts!" Instead, say, "I want to be touched this way" and then show them how you want to be touched. Then, let them know how much that turns you on.

Remember your partner's pleasure by asking, "Does this feel good?" A sexy, "Tell me what you want" request can go a long way in allowing your partner to let you know what he or she would like to get more turned on, and can add to the excitement to the moment. Do not get too technical during sex though.

In fact, never discuss the logistics of sex in the bedroom if you feel it will leave your partner feeling anything other than turned on. Your partner is way too vulnerable during sex, and the last thing you want to do is to increase performance anxiety.

If you must criticize your partner, do it in neutral territory, at a non-sexual time. For instance, talk to your partner at the kitchen table when relaxing over a hot beverage. Then, be very careful to compliment, then request. Or, explain the situation without blaming. An example would be, "It irritates my clit when it is stimulated too long or too hard, I would like to experience light touches, with not as much time spent on that spot."

When you build your partner up, avoid blaming and keep anything other than tantalizing sex talk out of the bedroom, your partner will feel better about sex and will be able to relax. Not only will relaxation help your partner enjoy sex more, but he or she will be more open to experimenting and really letting loose in ways that will increase your enjoyment as well.

Conclusion

By reading the "WOW Orgasms: A Sex Guide to Make a Pleasure Explosion in Bed", you now have all the knowledge to become a world class lover. Not only that, but you know exactly what to do to create the most powerful and exquisite orgasms, for yourself and your partner.

Remember how important sex is and set a goal to have it at least three or four times a week. Even a quickie counts for sex, but schedule at least an hour or more as often as possible to spend naked time with your lover. Also, take a break every so often for three to four days in order to build up for the most intense orgasms.

Follow the WOW Sex formula for the best sex and orgasms of your entire life:

- Get 20 minutes of cardio and at least 10 minutes of yoga or other stretching exercises per day.

- Eat healthy foods, and choose foods for how they increase your sexual pleasure.

- Build mindfulness skills to be able to stay fully in the moment. Also, lighten up and enjoy sex with a sense of playfulness and adventure.

- Take time to relax, exfoliate, and otherwise pamper yourself.

- Pursue foreplay early and often.

- Experiment with different ways of having sex, such as different positions and different types of stimulation in order to achieve heightened pleasure.

-   Enjoy the most powerful orgasms of your life.

-   Keep an open and positive line of communication with your partner.

Best wishes for an amazing sex life!